INTRODUCTION

THE STAIRS DIET progressively adds changes to your eating routine over a three month period. Just as a person takes one step at a time up a flight of stairs, each week you will take one step toward better health. **THE STAIRS DIET** does not require you to purchase expensive foods or food processing equipment. **THE STAIRS DIET** will save time on cooking. **THE STAIRS DIET** will reduce your weekly food cost. **THE STAIRS DIET** will change your life. **THE STAIRS DIET** is not a book. **THE STAIRS DIET** is an instruction manual. No fluff, no pictures, no testimonials. When you get an instruction manual for a piece of furniture do you need pictures and unnecessary information about what type of wood the table is made out of? No. This is an instruction manual for your health, for you future, for your life. Your time is too precious to waste. You will see how easy **THE STAIRS DIET** is to follow and more importantly you will see results.

WHY MOST DIETS DON'T WORK

Technically, they are not even diets. The idea of a diet has been misunderstood for years. Most people understand a diet to be an eating program that helps you lose weight. That is *NOT* what a diet is. By definition a diet is: food and drink regularly consumed, or simply put: habitual nourishment. Now ask yourself, are you going to habitually drink *only* juice for the rest of your life? Are you going to *only* eat cabbage soup everyday for the rest of your life? Are you going to eat *only* bananas, or cut out carbs, or eat *only* "healthy" cookies everyday for the rest of your life? Let's call these so called "diets" what they really are; scams. It's time to take make healthy lifestyle changes. It's time for **THE STAIRS DIET.**

WHY THE STAIRS DIET WORKS

Most scam diets encourage people to make too many changes too quickly. Picture someone who eats a bagel, muffin or donut every morning. Then grabs a fast food lunch from the drive-thru. They finish the night with a delivered or frozen pizza. Maybe that someone is you. And oh yeah don't forget about the snacks during the day. The bag of chips, the candy bar and the energy drinks. Now imagine telling that person to change their whole eating routine, breakfast, lunch, dinner, and snacks all at once. Come on! Let's get serious! Even the person who does that for two or three weeks will eventually go back to their old habits. Sure they lost a few pounds, but what happened next. THE WEIGHT COMES BACK! You know them, you've seen them, don't be them. If you want to be a shapeshifter, losing and gaining weight in a repetitive cycle, then go with one of those scam diets. But if you want to actually change your health, **THE STAIRS DIET** is the way to go.

WEEK 2

EAT 2 BOILED EGGS EVERY MORNING

MONDAY   TUESDAY   WEDNESDAY   THURSDAY   FRIDAY   SATURDAY   SUNDAY

EAT 1 APPLE A DAY

MONDAY   TUESDAY   WEDNESDAY   THURSDAY   FRIDAY   SATURDAY   SUNDAY

An apple a day keeps the doctor away. How many times have you heard this? Do you believe it? Then do it. You don't need to know the science behind how an apple break down as it travels through your digestive system. If you know it's good for you, eat it. For one week eat an apple everyday. It doesn't matter what time you eat it. Simply eat an apple everyday. Simple right? That's why it's the first step. There are over 7,000 types of apples in the world. 7,000! In your grocery store there are probably at least 10 types of apples. So there is no excuse why you should not be able to find at least 1 type of apple that you enjoy. I've heard excuses why people don't eat apples. "I don't like eating apples when they're cold". Then leave them out on the counter. "I don't like biting into an apple, it hurts my teeth" Then cut it up. Here is the best part about this first step. You don't have to change anything else in your diet this week. You can drink soda, eat donuts and candy, you can even go to the fast food drive thru, but make sure....you eat 1 apple every day.

WEEK 1

EAT 1 APPLE A DAY

MONDAY   TUESDAY   WEDNESDAY   THURSDAY   FRIDAY   SATURDAY   SUNDAY

THE PROCESS

The left side of the page list the steps that are to be followed that week. Below each step is a list of the weekdays. Mark each day you complete the step. On the right side of the page you will find commentary about the new step of the week. The step for the week is to be followed for that week and all the weeks that follow. For example, the step for week 1 will be followed week 1. Week 2 you will continue to follow the week 1 step *and* follow the step for week 2. Week 3 you will follow the steps from weeks 1 and 2 as well as the week 3 step, and so on and so forth. Got it? Great! Let's Begin.

In 2016 the oldest woman in the world turned 117. She said she eats 2 eggs a day and has done so for the previous 90 years. Enough said right? Amazing! How do you like your eggs? How many times have you been asked that at a restaurant? Everytime you go to breakfast. But here's the thing. Who has time to scramble, poach or fry two eggs every morning. Not most of us. But we all have time to boil them. Here's why you will love this step. Because you can be lazy and complete it. Get a pack of 18 eggs and boil 9 eggs at a time. This will cover you for 3 days (2 eggs each morning), with one extra egg. You will find out what to do with the extra egg in week 3. Boiling 9 eggs at a time also helps the eggs stay fresher. Boil the eggs for 20 minutes. Set a timer so that you know when the eggs are done. When the eggs have cooled down, take the eggs out of the shells and put them in sealable sandwich bags 2 eggs per bag. Put them in the fridge and you're set for the next few mornings. You don't have to prepare breakfast in the morning, but you should have it prepared for the morning. You can boil your eggs at night or whenever it's convenient for you. The nice thing about this step and all steps that follow is that the foods are easy to take with you. You can heat the eggs up at work or eat them cold on your morning drive. The goal is to eat a healthy breakfast while saving time and money. Oh yeah, that's right, I forgot to mention, no more drive-thru breakfast stops. You can still go to the drive thru for lunch, eat your frozen pizza for dinner, and drink your soda. Just don't forget to grab your 2 eggs in the morning.

WEEK 3

EAT A SPINACH SALAD TWICE A WEEK FOR DINNER

MONDAY   TUESDAY   WEDNESDAY   THURSDAY   FRIDAY   SATURDAY   SUNDAY

EAT 2 BOILED EGGS EVERY MORNING

MONDAY   TUESDAY   WEDNESDAY   THURSDAY   FRIDAY   SATURDAY   SUNDAY

EAT 1 APPLE A DAY

MONDAY   TUESDAY   WEDNESDAY   THURSDAY   FRIDAY   SATURDAY   SUNDAY

So by now you are boiling your eggs twice a week. That's great. But you boil 9 at a time and eat 2 each morning. What do you do with the 9th egg? Put it in your spinach salad. Spinach is great for you. Spinach can also be bought in pre-washed bags and ready to eat. Quick, cheap and easy. You will see this is a recurring theme with **THE STAIRS DIET**. Quick, cheap and easy. But you're going to want to add a little extra to that salad. Thankfully you have been buying apples for the past two weeks. Why not cut up half of an apple and put it in your salad. Or you could add another fruit (pears, strawberry, blueberry). Don't forget to include pecans or walnuts and maybe a little feta cheese. You may want to drizzle some honey over your salad and finish it off with a nice Raspberry Vinaigrette or salad dressing of your choice. Experiment until you find a mixture that you can eat two times per week.

WEEK 4

DRINK 1/3 OF A GALLON OF WATER A DAY

MONDAY   TUESDAY   WEDNESDAY   THURSDAY   FRIDAY   SATURDAY   SUNDAY

EAT A SPINACH SALAD TWICE A WEEK FOR DINNER

MONDAY   TUESDAY   WEDNESDAY   THURSDAY   FRIDAY   SATURDAY   SUNDAY

EAT 2 BOILED EGGS EVERY MORNING

MONDAY   TUESDAY   WEDNESDAY   THURSDAY   FRIDAY   SATURDAY   SUNDAY

EAT 1 APPLE A DAY

MONDAY   TUESDAY   WEDNESDAY   THURSDAY   FRIDAY   SATURDAY   SUNDAY

Drinking ⅓ of a gallon of water may sound like a lot. But it's not. Look at it this way. Would you consider drinking (3) 16.9 ounce bottles of water in a day a lot? No way! That is ⅓ of a gallon of water. Those 3 bottles of water don't even equal 64 ounces, which is what many sources recommend we drink per day. You gotta love **THE STAIRS DIET**. You can still drink your soda, coffee and energy drinks. As long as you drink 3 bottles of water per day you're good to go. It would be good to pick up a 24 or 36 pack of 16.9 ounce water bottles. This way you are set for the week(s). Leave some in your car, some in the refrigerator at work, or at your desk and some at your house. Of course you can drink more water than that each day if you'd like. Three bottles is simply the minimum...for now. The problem with scam diets is that they often want you to stop drinking soda and energy drinks immediately. While going cold turkey may work for some. The chances of a relapse back to these sugary drinks is more likely. So enjoy your soda, enjoy your energy drink, but make sure you drink your (3) 16.9 ounce water bottles each day.

WEEK 5

EAT CHICKEN WITH VEGETABLES 3 TIMES A WEEK

MONDAY   TUESDAY   WEDNESDAY   THURSDAY   FRIDAY   SATURDAY   SUNDAY

DRINK 1/3 OF A GALLON OF WATER A DAY

MONDAY   TUESDAY   WEDNESDAY   THURSDAY   FRIDAY   SATURDAY   SUNDAY

EAT A SPINACH SALAD TWICE A WEEK FOR DINNER

MONDAY   TUESDAY   WEDNESDAY   THURSDAY   FRIDAY   SATURDAY   SUNDAY

EAT 2 BOILED EGGS EVERY MORNING

MONDAY   TUESDAY   WEDNESDAY   THURSDAY   FRIDAY   SATURDAY   SUNDAY

EAT 1 APPLE A DAY

MONDAY   TUESDAY   WEDNESDAY   THURSDAY   FRIDAY   SATURDAY   SUNDAY

Chicken is one of the most common meats eaten around the world. You however, probably don't have time to bake, fillet, or fry chicken 3 times a week. Actually, you should never fry chicken, but that's a whole nother topic. What you can do is buy a ready to go rotisserie chicken from the store and eat portions of *it* 3 times a week. You will want to accompany the chicken with vegetables. Get a pack of frozen vegetables (preferably green vegetables such as broccoli, asparagus or brussel sprouts) and heat it up in the microwave. Some people say that microwave vegetables are bad for you. Don't believe them. How can vegetables be bad for you? If you want something more to accompany this meal you can heat up a minute rice in the microwave. So just to recap: Pick up a ready to go chicken on your way home, eat it for dinner along with vegetables and rice. Pack a portion for lunch the next day and then have it for dinner the next night.

WEEK 6

EAT ALMONDS WITH YOUR APPLE (THE A TEAM)

MONDAY   TUESDAY   WEDNESDAY   THURSDAY   FRIDAY   SATURDAY   SUNDAY

EAT CHICKEN WITH VEGETABLES 3 TIMES A WEEK

MONDAY   TUESDAY   WEDNESDAY   THURSDAY   FRIDAY   SATURDAY   SUNDAY

DRINK 1/3 OF A GALLON OF WATER A DAY

MONDAY   TUESDAY   WEDNESDAY   THURSDAY   FRIDAY   SATURDAY   SUNDAY

EAT A SPINACH SALAD TWICE A WEEK FOR DINNER

MONDAY   TUESDAY   WEDNESDAY   THURSDAY   FRIDAY   SATURDAY   SUNDAY

EAT 2 BOILED EGGS EVERY MORNING

MONDAY   TUESDAY   WEDNESDAY   THURSDAY   FRIDAY   SATURDAY   SUNDAY

EAT 1 APPLE A DAY

MONDAY   TUESDAY   WEDNESDAY   THURSDAY   FRIDAY   SATURDAY   SUNDAY

At this point you're doing great. You're eating your apple, eating your eggs and drinking your ⅓ gallon of water everyday. Along with the other steps of course. So now you are going to add almonds into the mix. Almonds are great for you. No need to go into grave detail about that. Almonds are also great with apples. When you eat your apple add a handful of almonds. Make sure that you don't eat so many almonds that you are unable to finish the apple. You need to balance the two. Allow them to work together as a team. The A Team. Another thing to think about is when you eat The A Team. Make The A Team your first snack of the day. After you have eaten your eggs and you start to feel hungry again, it's time for The A Team. It will probably be time for a bathroom break soon thereafter. Let's go ahead and address that now. You've probably noticed that you're using the bathroom a few more times each day since starting **THE STAIRS DIET**. Your body's just letting you know that everything's working properly. Keep up the good work.

WEEK 7

EAT 1 BANANA A DAY WITH PEANUTS

MONDAY   TUESDAY   WEDNESDAY   THURSDAY   FRIDAY   SATURDAY   SUNDAY

EAT ALMONDS WITH YOUR APPLE (THE A TEAM)

MONDAY   TUESDAY   WEDNESDAY   THURSDAY   FRIDAY   SATURDAY   SUNDAY

EAT CHICKEN WITH VEGETABLES 3 TIMES A WEEK

MONDAY   TUESDAY   WEDNESDAY   THURSDAY   FRIDAY   SATURDAY   SUNDAY

DRINK 1/3 OF A GALLON OF WATER A DAY

MONDAY   TUESDAY   WEDNESDAY   THURSDAY   FRIDAY   SATURDAY   SUNDAY

EAT A SPINACH SALAD TWICE A WEEK FOR DINNER

MONDAY   TUESDAY   WEDNESDAY   THURSDAY   FRIDAY   SATURDAY   SUNDAY

EAT 2 BOILED EGGS EVERY MORNING

MONDAY   TUESDAY   WEDNESDAY   THURSDAY   FRIDAY   SATURDAY   SUNDAY

EAT 1 APPLE A DAY

MONDAY   TUESDAY   WEDNESDAY   THURSDAY   FRIDAY   SATURDAY   SUNDAY

Bananas are great for you. If you know something is good for you, you should...eat it. Eat your banana as an afternoon snack. Eat your banana with peanuts. Salted, dry roasted or honey roasted are all great options. If you don't like peanuts you can eat cashews, walnuts, pecans or more almonds with your banana.

STAIRS DIET TIP: ALWAYS HAVE SNACKS ON HAND. Some people only pack enough snacks for that day, but wouldn't it be much wiser and easier to have snacks at multiple locations. Especially if you're going to be eating the same snacks each day. Have almonds, peanuts, walnuts, or whatever nut you decide to eat regularly in your car, at your job,, and at home at all times. So buy in bulk and distribute accordingly. This way you're always prepared. Always having snacks on hand will make it easy to stick to your **THE STAIRS DIET** when you're tempted to eat unhealthy foods.

WEEK 8

DON'T EAT AFTER 8PM

MONDAY   TUESDAY   WEDNESDAY   THURSDAY   FRIDAY   SATURDAY   SUNDAY

EAT 1 BANANA A DAY WITH PEANUTS

MONDAY   TUESDAY   WEDNESDAY   THURSDAY   FRIDAY   SATURDAY   SUNDAY

EAT ALMONDS WITH YOUR APPLE (THE A TEAM)

MONDAY   TUESDAY   WEDNESDAY   THURSDAY   FRIDAY   SATURDAY   SUNDAY

EAT CHICKEN WITH VEGETABLES 3 TIMES A WEEK

MONDAY   TUESDAY   WEDNESDAY   THURSDAY   FRIDAY   SATURDAY   SUNDAY

DRINK 1/3 OF A GALLON OF WATER A DAY

MONDAY   TUESDAY   WEDNESDAY   THURSDAY   FRIDAY   SATURDAY   SUNDAY

EAT A SPINACH SALAD TWICE A WEEK FOR DINNER

MONDAY   TUESDAY   WEDNESDAY   THURSDAY   FRIDAY   SATURDAY   SUNDAY

EAT 2 BOILED EGGS EVERY MORNING

MONDAY   TUESDAY   WEDNESDAY   THURSDAY   FRIDAY   SATURDAY   SUNDAY

EAT 1 APPLE A DAY

MONDAY   TUESDAY   WEDNESDAY   THURSDAY   FRIDAY   SATURDAY   SUNDAY

How appropriate for this step to fall on the 8th week. You know that eating late is horrible for you. So don't do it. This step is not about choosing healthy options. It's about being self disciplined. Since you're not going to be eating late you can go to bed early. This means you will wake up early. With this extra time in the morning you can exercise, read and make sure you have your snacks and lunch for the day.

WEEK 9

DRINK 2/3 OF A GALLON OF WATER A DAY

MONDAY   TUESDAY   WEDNESDAY   THURSDAY   FRIDAY   SATURDAY   SUNDAY

DON'T EAT AFTER 8 PM

MONDAY   TUESDAY   WEDNESDAY   THURSDAY   FRIDAY   SATURDAY   SUNDAY

EAT 1 BANANA A DAY WITH PEANUTS

MONDAY   TUESDAY   WEDNESDAY   THURSDAY   FRIDAY   SATURDAY   SUNDAY

EAT ALMONDS WITH YOUR APPLE (THE A TEAM)

MONDAY   TUESDAY   WEDNESDAY   THURSDAY   FRIDAY   SATURDAY   SUNDAY

EAT CHICKEN WITH VEGETABLES 3 TIMES A WEEK

MONDAY   TUESDAY   WEDNESDAY   THURSDAY   FRIDAY   SATURDAY   SUNDAY

EAT A SPINACH SALAD TWICE A WEEK FOR DINNER

MONDAY   TUESDAY   WEDNESDAY   THURSDAY   FRIDAY   SATURDAY   SUNDAY

EAT 2 BOILED EGGS EVERY MORNING

MONDAY   TUESDAY   WEDNESDAY   THURSDAY   FRIDAY   SATURDAY   SUNDAY

EAT 1 APPLE A DAY

MONDAY   TUESDAY   WEDNESDAY   THURSDAY   FRIDAY   SATURDAY   SUNDAY

All the weeks prior to this week you have been drinking your (3) 16.9 ounce bottles of water and now it's time to up that amount to (5) 16.9 ounce bottles of water. Which is roughly 2/3 of a gallon of water. In addition to that you want to limit the soda, juice, and energy drinks that you are consuming. You can continue to drink them, but the goal is to (spoiler alert) eliminate them completely. Don't let that thought scare you. You can do it. You've already begun to increase your desire for water. Let's keep that going.

STAIRS DIET TIP: Drink 1 water bottle (16.9 ounce) as soon as you wake up. The *FIRST* thing you do. Every night when you sleep your body loses water due to sweating, tossing and turning, and just from breathing. While the amount of water loss varies for each person, this fact is the same for everyone: You need to rehydrate yourself. And since you need to drink 5 (16.9 ounce) bottles of water, why not get started right away.

WEEK 10

EAT FISH 3 TIMES A WEEK (OR CHICKEN 3 MORE TIMES)

MONDAY   TUESDAY   WEDNESDAY   THURSDAY   FRIDAY   SATURDAY   SUNDAY

DRINK 2/3 OF A GALLON OF WATER A DAY

MONDAY   TUESDAY   WEDNESDAY   THURSDAY   FRIDAY   SATURDAY   SUNDAY

DON'T EAT AFTER 8PM

MONDAY   TUESDAY   WEDNESDAY   THURSDAY   FRIDAY   SATURDAY   SUNDAY

EAT 1 BANANA A DAY WITH PEANUTS

MONDAY   TUESDAY   WEDNESDAY   THURSDAY   FRIDAY   SATURDAY   SUNDAY

EAT ALMONDS WITH YOUR APPLE (THE A TEAM)

MONDAY   TUESDAY   WEDNESDAY   THURSDAY   FRIDAY   SATURDAY   SUNDAY

EAT CHICKEN WITH VEGETABLES 3 TIMES A WEEK

MONDAY   TUESDAY   WEDNESDAY   THURSDAY   FRIDAY   SATURDAY   SUNDAY

EAT A SPINACH SALAD TWICE A WEEK FOR DINNER

MONDAY   TUESDAY   WEDNESDAY   THURSDAY   FRIDAY   SATURDAY   SUNDAY

EAT 2 BOILED EGGS EVERY MORNING

MONDAY   TUESDAY   WEDNESDAY   THURSDAY   FRIDAY   SATURDAY   SUNDAY

EAT 1 APPLE A DAY

MONDAY   TUESDAY   WEDNESDAY   THURSDAY   FRIDAY   SATURDAY   SUNDAY

Fish is great for you, and easy to cook. Take salmon for example. A little olive oil, salt, and pepper, bake it for 35 minutes and you're done. You could do the same thing with cod or tilapia. Of course not everybody likes fish. If you are one of those people substitute a ready to go rotisserie chicken or ready to go turkey instead. The side dishes that go with this step are the same as the Week 5 Step. Add microwave vegetables and rice to accompany your main course.

WEEK 11

EAT FAST FOOD 2 TIMES A WEEK – THAT'S RIGHT FAST FOOD

MONDAY   TUESDAY   WEDNESDAY   THURSDAY   FRIDAY   SATURDAY   SUNDAY

EAT FISH 3 TIMES A WEEK (OR CHICKEN 3 MORE TIMES)

MONDAY   TUESDAY   WEDNESDAY   THURSDAY   FRIDAY   SATURDAY   SUNDAY

DRINK 2/3 OF A GALLON OF WATER A DAY

MONDAY   TUESDAY   WEDNESDAY   THURSDAY   FRIDAY   SATURDAY   SUNDAY

DON'T EAT AFTER 8PM

MONDAY   TUESDAY   WEDNESDAY   THURSDAY   FRIDAY   SATURDAY   SUNDAY

EAT 1 BANANA A DAY WITH PEANUTS

MONDAY   TUESDAY   WEDNESDAY   THURSDAY   FRIDAY   SATURDAY   SUNDAY

EAT ALMONDS WITH YOUR APPLE (THE A TEAM)

MONDAY   TUESDAY   WEDNESDAY   THURSDAY   FRIDAY   SATURDAY   SUNDAY

EAT CHICKEN WITH VEGETABLES 3 TIMES A WEEK

MONDAY   TUESDAY   WEDNESDAY   THURSDAY   FRIDAY   SATURDAY   SUNDAY

EAT A SPINACH SALAD TWICE A WEEK FOR DINNER

MONDAY   TUESDAY   WEDNESDAY   THURSDAY   FRIDAY   SATURDAY   SUNDAY

EAT 2 BOILED EGGS EVERY MORNING

MONDAY   TUESDAY   WEDNESDAY   THURSDAY   FRIDAY   SATURDAY   SUNDAY

EAT 1 APPLE A DAY

MONDAY   TUESDAY   WEDNESDAY   THURSDAY   FRIDAY   SATURDAY   SUNDAY

If you're thinking there must be a catch, you're right, there is. Yes you can eat fast food twice a week, but from where? The grocery store, that's where! Here's what you do. Visit the deli section of your local grocery store. Choose a healthy salad that has meat in it. Most grocery stores are going to have at least 1 type of chicken salad, but probably even more chicken salad options than that. The first time you go you may have to sample a few to find out which salads you like, but on every visit after that you can go in quickly and pick the salad you want and the amount you want. What about a side dish? You're going to love this. Grab a bag of potato chips. Yes potato chips! Not just any chips though. Make sure you choose a brand that has only 3 ingredients. That may sound difficult, but there are actually lots of brands that only use potatoes, oil, and salt. And there are lots of chip varieties to choose from: sweet potato, apple, parsnips, beets. The initial process of choosing your favorite meat salad and bag of chips will take a while, but after that you should be in and out of the grocery store in less than eight minutes. Maybe you decide to run to the grocery store on your lunch break or maybe on the weekends while you're out running errands. Whatever the case, this is your new version of FAST FOOD. Bonappetit!

WEEK 12

DRINK 1 GALLON OF WATER EVERYDAY

MONDAY   TUESDAY   WEDNESDAY   THURSDAY   FRIDAY   SATURDAY   SUNDAY

EAT FAST FOOD 2 TIMES A WEEK - THAT'S RIGHT FAST FOOD

MONDAY   TUESDAY   WEDNESDAY   THURSDAY   FRIDAY   SATURDAY   SUNDAY

EAT FISH 3 TIMES A WEEK (OR CHICKEN 3 MORE TIMES)

MONDAY   TUESDAY   WEDNESDAY   THURSDAY   FRIDAY   SATURDAY   SUNDAY

STOP EATING AFTER 8PM

MONDAY   TUESDAY   WEDNESDAY   THURSDAY   FRIDAY   SATURDAY   SUNDAY

EAT 1 BANANA A DAY WITH PEANUTS

MONDAY   TUESDAY   WEDNESDAY   THURSDAY   FRIDAY   SATURDAY   SUNDAY

EAT ALMONDS WITH YOUR APPLE (THE A TEAM)

MONDAY   TUESDAY   WEDNESDAY   THURSDAY   FRIDAY   SATURDAY   SUNDAY

EAT CHICKEN WITH VEGETABLES 3 TIMES A WEEK

MONDAY   TUESDAY   WEDNESDAY   THURSDAY   FRIDAY   SATURDAY   SUNDAY

EAT A SPINACH SALAD TWICE A WEEK FOR DINNER

MONDAY   TUESDAY   WEDNESDAY   THURSDAY   FRIDAY   SATURDAY   SUNDAY

EAT 2 BOILED EGGS EVERY MORNING

MONDAY   TUESDAY   WEDNESDAY   THURSDAY   FRIDAY   SATURDAY   SUNDAY

EAT 1 APPLE A DAY

MONDAY   TUESDAY   WEDNESDAY   THURSDAY   FRIDAY   SATURDAY   SUNDAY

A gallon of water is only (8) 16.9 water bottles per day. When you put it that way it sounds much easier than saying drink a gallon of water a day. How you do it is up to you. You could label the water bottles 1 thru 8 on the bottle tops and drink them throughout the day (Including your first bottle as soon as you wake up). If you work from home you could simply take 1 gallon for each day and write the days of the week on them. You could divide the gallon of water amongst several sports bottles that equal 1 gallon. Whatever works best for you. You can drink more than 1 gallon a day, and by this point you may have developed such a thirst for water that you want to drink more than that. It's all you will be drinking from now on anyway. That's right! From this point forward, no more soda, juice, or energy drinks, EVER! Isn't it so much easier, quicker, cheaper and healthier to drink more water anyway.

CONCLUSION

Congratulations on completing **THE STAIRS DIET**. This is not the end however. Perhaps over the course of these steps you have thought of additional steps you would like to take. By all means keep climbing, step by step. You also noticed that **THE STAIRS DIET** does not cover every single meal of the week. **THE STAIRS DIET** is the basis of your diet. No doubt you will go out to eat with friends and go to various parties for the rest of your life. But now you will make healthy decisions because that has become your pattern, your routine, your diet.